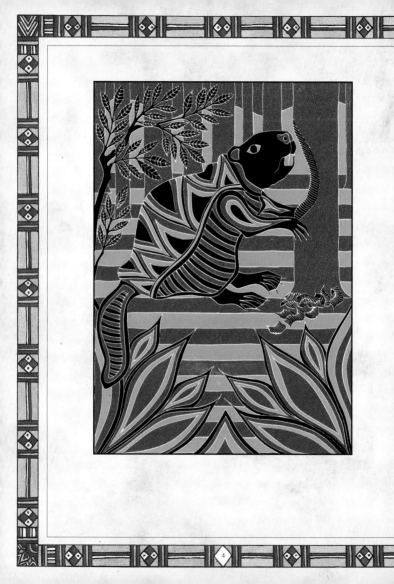

THE LITTLE LIBRARY OF EARTH MEDICINE

BEAVER

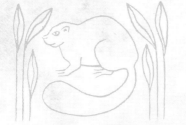

Kenneth Meadows

Illustrations by Jo Donegan

DORLING KINDERSLEY
LONDON • NEW YORK • SYDNEY • MOSCOW

A DORLING KINDERSLEY BOOK

Managing editor: Jonathan Metcalf
Managing art editor: Peter Cross
Production manager: Michelle Thomas

The Little Library of Earth Medicine was
produced, edited and designed by
GLS Editorial and Design
Garden Studios, 11-15 Betterton Street
London WC2H 9BP

GLS Editorial and Design
Editorial director: Jane Laing
Design director: Ruth Shane
Project designer: Luke Herriott
Editors: Claire Calman, Terry Burrows, Victoria Sorzano

Additional illustrations: Roy Flooks 16, 17, 31; John Lawrence 38
Special photography: Mark Hamilton
Picture credits: American Natural History Museum 8-9, 12, 14-15, 32

First published in Great Britain in 1998
by Dorling Kindersley Limited
9 Henrietta Street, London WC2E 8PS

2 4 6 8 10 9 7 5 3 1

A CIP catalogue record for this book is available from the British Library

UK ISBN 0 7513 0515 4   AUSTRALIAN ISBN 1 86466 032 5

Reproduced by Kestrel Digital Colour Ltd, Chelmsford, Essex
Printed and bound in Hong Kong by Imago

CONTENTS

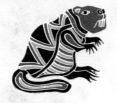

INTRODUCING
EARTH MEDICINE

To Native Americans, medicine is not an external
substance but an inner power that is found in
both Nature and ourselves.

E arth Medicine is a unique
method of personality
profiling that draws on
Native American under-
standing of the Universe; and
on the principles embodied in
sacred Medicine Wheels.

Native Americans believed
that spirit, although invisible,
permeated Nature, so that
everything in Nature was
sacred. Animals were
perceived as acting as

Shaman's rattle
*Shamans used rattles to connect
with their inner spirit. This is a
Tlingit shaman's wooden rattle.*

messengers of spirit. They
also appeared in waking
dreams to impart power
known as "medicine". The
recipients of such dreams
honoured the animal
species that appeared to
them by rendering their
images on ceremonial and
everyday artefacts.

NATURE WITHIN SELF
Native American shamans
– tribal wisemen –
recognized similarities
between the natural forces
prevalent during the seasons and
the characteristics of those born

*"Spirit has provided you with an opportunity to
study in Nature's university."* Stoney teaching

during corresponding times of the year. They also noted how personality is affected by the four phases of the Moon – at birth and throughout life – and by the continual alternation of energy flow, from active to passive. This view is encapsulated in Earth Medicine, which helps you to recognize how the dynamics of Nature function within you and how the potential strengths you were born with can be developed.

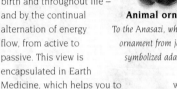

Animal ornament
To the Anasazi, who carved this ornament from jet, the frog symbolized adaptability.

MEDICINE WHEELS

Native American cultural traditions embrace a variety of circular symbolic images and objects. These sacred hoops have become known as Medicine

Feast dish
Stylized bear carvings adorn this Tlingit feast dish. To the American Indian, the bear symbolizes strength and self-sufficiency.

Wheels, due to their similarity to the spoked wheels of the wagons that carried settlers into the heartlands of once-Native American territory. Each Medicine Wheel showed how different objects or qualities related to one another within the context of a greater whole, and how different forces and energies moved within it.

One Medicine Wheel might be regarded as the master wheel because it indicated balance within Nature and the most effective way of achieving harmony with the Universe and ourselves. It is upon this master Medicine Wheel (see pp.10–11) that Earth Medicine is structured.

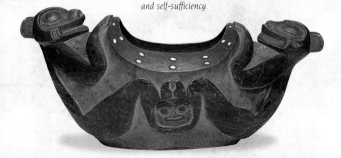

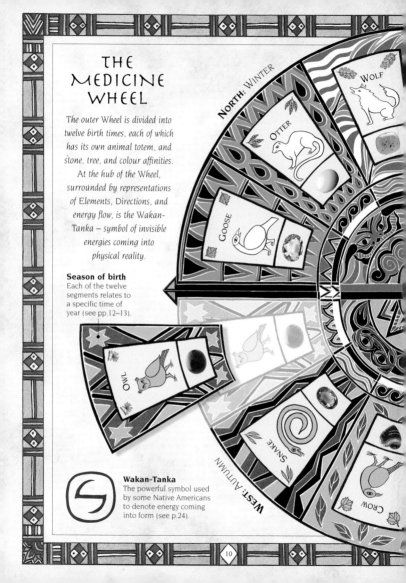

THE MEDICINE WHEEL

The outer Wheel is divided into twelve birth times, each of which has its own animal totem, and stone, tree, and colour affinities.

At the hub of the Wheel, surrounded by representations of Elements, Directions, and energy flow, is the Wakan-Tanka – symbol of invisible energies coming into physical reality.

Season of birth
Each of the twelve segments relates to a specific time of year (see pp.12–13).

Wakan-Tanka
The powerful symbol used by some Native Americans to denote energy coming into form (see p.24).

NORTH: WINTER

WEST: AUTUMN

WOLF

OTTER

GOOSE

OWL

SNAKE

CROW

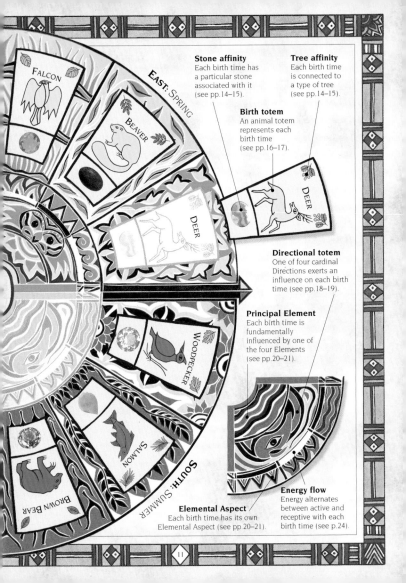

Stone affinity
Each birth time has a particular stone associated with it (see pp.14–15).

Tree affinity
Each birth time is connected to a type of tree (see pp.14–15).

Birth totem
An animal totem represents each birth time (see pp.16–17).

FALCON

EAST: SPRING

BEAVER

DEER

DEER

Directional totem
One of four cardinal Directions exerts an influence on each birth time (see pp.18–19).

Principal Element
Each birth time is fundamentally influenced by one of the four Elements (see pp.20–21).

WOODPECKER

SALMON

BROWN BEAR

SOUTH: SUMMER

Energy flow
Energy alternates between active and receptive with each birth time (see p.24).

Elemental Aspect
Each birth time has its own Elemental Aspect (see pp.20–21).

THE TWELVE
BIRTH TIMES

THE STRUCTURE OF THE MEDICINE WHEEL IS BASED UPON THE SEASONS TO REFLECT THE POWERFUL INFLUENCE OF NATURE ON HUMAN PERSONALITY.

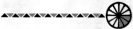

The Medicine Wheel classifies human nature into twelve personality types, each corresponding to the characteristics of Nature at a particular time of the year. It is designed to act as a kind of map to help you discover your strengths and weaknesses, your inner drives and instinctive behaviours, and your true potential.

The four seasons form the basis of the Wheel's structure, with the Summer and Winter solstices and the Spring and Autumn equinoxes marking each season's passing. In Earth Medicine,

each season is a metaphor for a stage of human growth and development. Spring is likened to infancy and the newness of life; and Summer to the exuberance of youth and of rapid development. Autumn represents the fulfilment that mature adulthood brings, while Winter symbolizes the accumulated wisdom that can be drawn upon in later life.

Each seasonal quarter of the Wheel is further divided into three periods, making twelve time segments altogether. The time of your birth determines the direction from which

Seasonal rites

Performers at the Iroquois mid-Winter ceremony wore masks made of braided maize husks. They danced to attune themselves to energies that would ensure a good harvest.

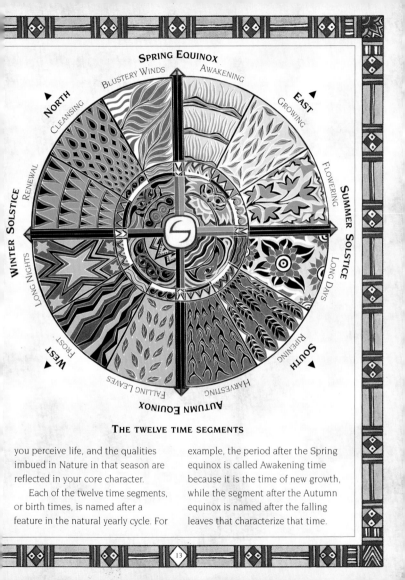

THE TWELVE TIME SEGMENTS

you perceive life, and the qualities imbued in Nature in that season are reflected in your core character.

Each of the twelve time segments, or birth times, is named after a feature in the natural yearly cycle. For example, the period after the Spring equinox is called Awakening time because it is the time of new growth, while the segment after the Autumn equinox is named after the falling leaves that characterize that time.

THE SIGNIFICANCE OF
TOTEMS

NATIVE AMERICANS BELIEVED THAT TOTEMS — ANIMAL
SYMBOLS — REPRESENTED ESSENTIAL TRUTHS AND ACTED
AS CONNECTIONS TO NATURAL POWERS.

A totem is an animal or natural object adopted as an emblem to typify certain distinctive qualities. Native Americans regarded animals, whose behaviour is predictable, as particularly useful guides to categorizing human patterns of behaviour.

A totem mirrors aspects of your nature and unlocks the intuitive knowledge that lies beyond the reasoning capacity of the intellect. It may take the form of a carving or moulding, a pictorial image, or a token of fur, feather, bone, tooth, or claw. Its presence serves as an immediate link with the energies it represents. A totem is therefore more effective than a glyph or symbol as an aid to comprehending non-physical powers and formative forces.

PRIMARY TOTEMS

In Earth Medicine you have three primary totems: a birth totem, a Directional totem, and an Elemental totem. Your *birth totem* is the embodiment of core characteristics that correspond with the dominant aspects of Nature during your birth time.

Symbol of strength

The handle of this Tlingit knife is carved with a raven and a bear head, symbols of insight and inner strength.

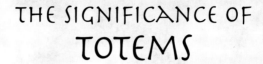

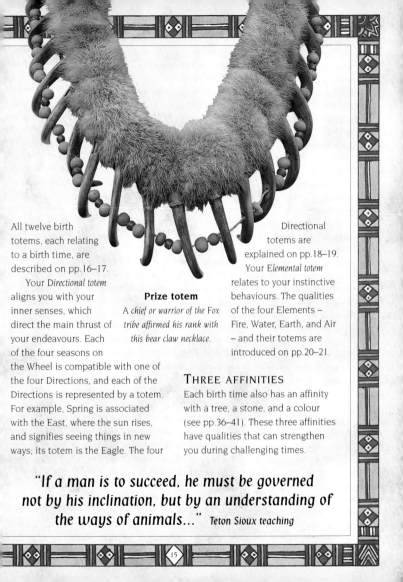

All twelve birth totems, each relating to a birth time, are described on pp.16–17.

Your *Directional totem* aligns you with your inner senses, which direct the main thrust of your endeavours. Each of the four seasons on the Wheel is compatible with one of the four Directions, and each of the Directions is represented by a totem. For example, Spring is associated with the East, where the sun rises, and signifies seeing things in new ways; its totem is the Eagle. The four

Prize totem

A chief or warrior of the Fox tribe affirmed his rank with this bear claw necklace.

Directional totems are explained on pp.18–19.

Your *Elemental totem* relates to your instinctive behaviours. The qualities of the four Elements – Fire, Water, Earth, and Air – and their totems are introduced on pp.20–21.

THREE AFFINITIES

Each birth time also has an affinity with a tree, a stone, and a colour (see pp.36–41). These three affinities have qualities that can strengthen you during challenging times.

"If a man is to succeed, he must be governed not by his inclination, but by an understanding of the ways of animals..." Teton Sioux teaching

THE TWELVE
BIRTH TOTEMS

THE TWELVE BIRTH TIMES ARE REPRESENTED BY TOTEMS,
EACH ONE AN ANIMAL THAT BEST EXPRESSES THE
QUALITIES INHERENT IN THAT BIRTH TIME.

Earth Medicine associates an animal totem with each birth time (the two sets of dates below reflect the difference in season between the northern and southern hemispheres). These animals help to connect you to the powers and abilities that they represent. For an in-depth study of the Beaver birth totem, see pp.28–29.

FALCON
21 March–19 April (N. Hem)
22 Sept–22 Oct (S. Hem)
Falcons are full of initiative, but often rush in to make decisions they may later regret. Lively and extroverted, they have enthusiasm for new experiences but can sometimes lack persistence.

DEER
21 May–20 June (N. Hem)
23 Nov–21 Dec (S. Hem)
Deer are willing to sacrifice the old for the new. They loathe routine, thriving on variety and challenges. They have a wild side, often leaping from one situation or relationship into another without reflection.

BEAVER
20 April–20 May (N. Hem)
23 Oct–22 Nov (S. Hem)
Practical and steady, Beavers have a capacity for perseverance. Good homemakers, they are warm and affectionate but need harmony and peace to avoid becoming irritable. They have a keen aesthetic sense.

WOODPECKER
21 June–21 July (N. Hem)
22 Dec–19 Jan (S. Hem)
Emotional and sensitive, Woodpeckers are warm to those closest to them, and willing to sacrifice their needs for those of their loved ones. They have lively imaginations but can be worriers.

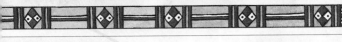

SALMON
22 July–21 August (N. Hem)
20 Jan–18 Feb (S. Hem)
Enthusiastic and self-confident,
Salmon people enjoy running things.
They are uncompromising and
forceful, and can occasionally seem a
little arrogant or self-important. They
are easily hurt by neglect.

OWL
23 Nov–21 Dec (N. Hem)
21 May–20 June (S. Hem)
Owls need freedom of expression.
They are lively, self-reliant, and have
an eye for detail. Inquisitive and
adaptable, they have a tendency to
overextend themselves. Owls are
often physically courageous.

BROWN BEAR
22 August–21 Sept (N. Hem)
19 Feb–20 March (S. Hem)
Brown Bears are hardworking,
practical, and self-reliant. They do
not like change, preferring to stick
to what is familiar. They have a flair
for fixing things, are good-natured,
and make good friends.

GOOSE
22 Dec–19 Jan (N. Hem)
21 June–21 July (S. Hem)
Goose people are far-sighted
idealists who are willing to explore
the unknown. They approach life with
enthusiasm, determined to fulfil their
dreams. They are perfectionists, and
can appear unduly serious.

CROW
22 Sept–22 Oct (N. Hem)
21 March–19 April (S. Hem)
Crows dislike solitude and feel most
comfortable in company. Although
usually pleasant and good-natured,
they can be strongly influenced by
negative atmospheres, becoming
gloomy and prickly.

OTTER
20 Jan–18 Feb (N. Hem)
22 July–21 August (S. Hem)
Otters are friendly, lively, and
perceptive. They feel inhibited by
too many rules and regulations,
which often makes them appear
eccentric. They like cleanliness and
order, and have original minds.

SNAKE
23 Oct–22 Nov (N. Hem)
20 April–20 May (S. Hem)
Snakes are secretive and
mysterious, hiding their feelings
beneath a cool exterior. Adaptable,
determined, and imaginative, they
are capable of bouncing back from
tough situations encountered in life.

WOLF
19 Feb–20 March (N. Hem)
22 August–21 Sept (S. Hem)
Wolves are sensitive, artistic, and
intuitive – people to whom others
turn for help. They value freedom
and their own space, and are easily
affected by others. They are
philosophical, trusting, and genuine.

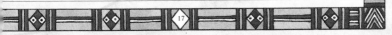

THE INFLUENCE OF THE
DIRECTIONS

ALSO KNOWN BY NATIVE AMERICANS AS THE FOUR
WINDS, THE INFLUENCE OF THE FOUR DIRECTIONS IS
EXPERIENCED THROUGH YOUR INNER SENSES.

Regarded as the "keepers" or "caretakers" of the Universe, the four Directions or alignments were also referred to by Native Americans as the four Winds because their presence was felt rather than seen.

DIRECTIONAL TOTEMS
In Earth Medicine, each Direction or Wind is associated with a season and a time of day. Thus the three Spring birth times – Awakening time, Growing time, and Flowering time –

all fall within the East Direction, and morning. The Direction to which your birth time belongs influences the nature of your inner senses.

The East Direction is associated with illumination. Its totem is the Eagle – a bird that soars close to the Sun and can see clearly from height. The South is the Direction of Summer and the afternoon. It signifies growth and fruition, fluidity, and emotions. Its totem, the Mouse, symbolizes productivity, feelings, and an ability to perceive detail.

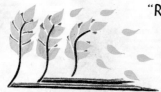

"Remember...the circle of the sky, the stars, the super-natural Winds breathing night and day...the four Directions." Pawnee teaching

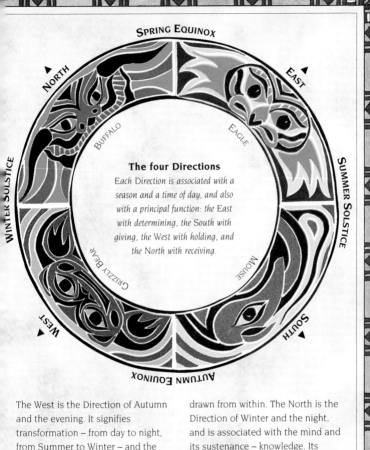

The four Directions

Each Direction is associated with a season and a time of day, and also with a principal function: the East with determining, the South with giving, the West with holding, and the North with receiving.

SPRING EQUINOX

NORTH

EAST

WINTER SOLSTICE

SUMMER SOLSTICE

WEST

SOUTH

AUTUMN EQUINOX

BUFFALO

EAGLE

GRIZZLY BEAR

MOUSE

The West is the Direction of Autumn and the evening. It signifies transformation – from day to night, from Summer to Winter – and the qualities of introspection and conservation. Its totem is the Grizzly Bear, which represents strength drawn from within. The North is the Direction of Winter and the night, and is associated with the mind and its sustenance – knowledge. Its totem is the Buffalo, an animal that was honoured by Native Americans as the great material "provider".

THE INFLUENCE OF THE ELEMENTS

THE FOUR ELEMENTS – AIR, FIRE, WATER, AND EARTH – PERVADE EVERYTHING AND INDICATE THE NATURE OF MOVEMENT AND THE ESSENCE OF WHO YOU ARE.

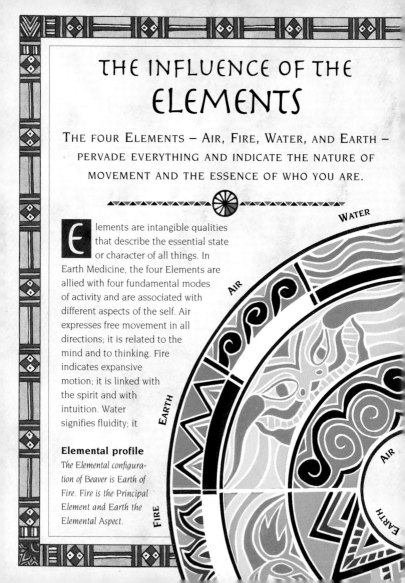

Elements are intangible qualities that describe the essential state or character of all things. In Earth Medicine, the four Elements are allied with four fundamental modes of activity and are associated with different aspects of the self. Air expresses free movement in all directions; it is related to the mind and to thinking. Fire indicates expansive motion; it is linked with the spirit and with intuition. Water signifies fluidity; it

Elemental profile

The Elemental configuration of Beaver is Earth of Fire. Fire is the Principal Element and Earth the Elemental Aspect.

WATER

AIR

EARTH

AIR

EARTH

FIRE

has associations with the soul and the emotions. Earth symbolizes stability; it is related to the physical body and the sensations.

ELEMENTAL DISTRIBUTION

On the Medicine Wheel one Element is associated with each of the four Directions – Fire in the East, Earth in the West, Air in the North, and Water in the South. These are known as the Principal Elements.

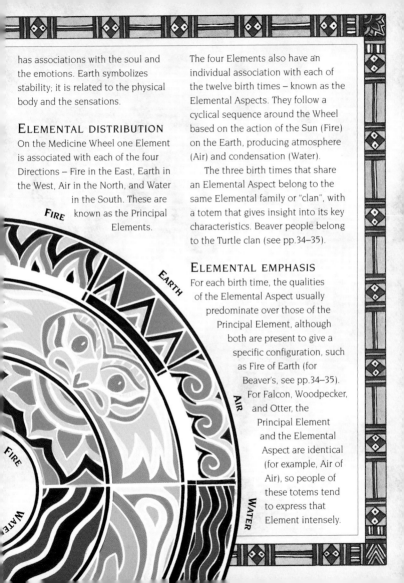

FIRE

EARTH

AIR

WATER

FIRE

WATER

The four Elements also have an individual association with each of the twelve birth times – known as the Elemental Aspects. They follow a cyclical sequence around the Wheel based on the action of the Sun (Fire) on the Earth, producing atmosphere (Air) and condensation (Water).

The three birth times that share an Elemental Aspect belong to the same Elemental family or "clan", with a totem that gives insight into its key characteristics. Beaver people belong to the Turtle clan (see pp.34–35).

ELEMENTAL EMPHASIS

For each birth time, the qualities of the Elemental Aspect usually predominate over those of the Principal Element, although both are present to give a specific configuration, such as Fire of Earth (for Beaver's, see pp.34–35). For Falcon, Woodpecker, and Otter, the Principal Element and the Elemental Aspect are identical (for example, Air of Air), so people of these totems tend to express that Element intensely.

THE INFLUENCE OF THE
MOON

THE WAXING AND WANING OF THE MOON DURING ITS
FOUR PHASES HAS A CRUCIAL INFLUENCE ON THE
FORMATION OF PERSONALITY AND HUMAN ENDEAVOUR.

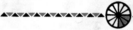

Native Americans regarded the Sun and Moon as indicators respectively of the active and receptive energies inherent in Nature (see p.24), as well as the measurers of time. They associated solar influences with conscious activity and the exercise of reason and the will, and lunar influences with subconscious activity and the emotional and intuitive aspects of human nature.

The Waxing Moon

This phase lasts for approximately eleven days. It is a time of growth and therefore ideal for developing new ideas and concentrating your efforts into new projects.

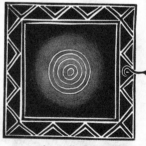

The Full Moon

Lasting about three days, this is when lunar power is at its height. It is therefore a good time for completing what was developed during the Waxing Moon.

THE FOUR PHASES

There are four phases in the twenty-nine-day lunar cycle, each one an expression of energy reflecting a particular mode of activity. They can be likened to the phases of growth of a flowering plant through the seasons: the emergence of buds (Waxing Moon), the bursting of flowers (Full Moon), the falling away of flowers (Waning Moon), and the germination of seeds (Dark Moon). The influence of each phase can be felt in two ways: in the formation of personality and in day-to-day life.

The energy expressed by the phase of the Moon at the time of your birth has a strong influence on personality. For instance, someone born during the Dark Moon is likely to be inward-looking, whilst a person born during the Full Moon may be more expressive. Someone born during a Waxing Moon is likely to have an outgoing nature, whilst a person born during a Waning Moon may be reserved. Consult a set of Moon tables to discover the phase the Moon was in on *your* birthday.

In your day-to-day life, the benefits of coming into harmony with the Moon's energies are considerable. Experience the energy of the four phases by consciously working with them. A Native American approach is described below.

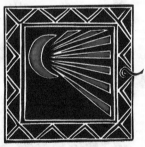

The Waning Moon
A time for making changes, this phase lasts for an average of eleven days. Use it to improve and modify, and to dispose of what is no longer needed or wanted.

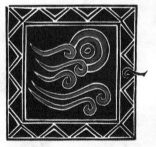

The Dark Moon
The Moon disappears from the sky for around four days. This is a time for contemplation of what has been achieved, and for germinating the seeds for the new.

THE INFLUENCE OF
ENERGY FLOW

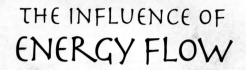

THE MEDICINE WHEEL REFLECTS THE PERFECT
BALANCE OF THE COMPLEMENTARY ACTIVE AND
RECEPTIVE ENERGIES THAT CO-EXIST IN NATURE.

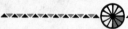

E nergy flows through Nature in two complementary ways, which can be expressed in terms of active and receptive, or male and female. The active energy principle is linked with the Elements of Fire and Air, and the receptive principle with Water and Earth.

Each of the twelve birth times has an active or receptive energy related to its Elemental Aspect. Travelling around the Wheel, the two energies alternate with each birth time, resulting in an equal balance of active and receptive energies, as in Nature.

Active energy is associated with the Sun and conscious activity. Those whose birth times take this principle prefer to pursue experience. They are conceptual,

energetic, outgoing, practical, and analytical. Receptive energy is associated with the Moon and subconscious activity. Those whose birth times take this principle prefer to attract experience. They are intuitive, reflective, conserving, emotional, and nurturing.

THE WAKAN-TANKA
At the heart of the Wheel lies an S-shape within a circle, the symbol of the life-giving source of everything that comes into physical existence – seemingly out of nothing. Named by the Plains Indians as Wakan-Tanka (Great Power), it can also be perceived as energy coming into form and form reverting to energy in the unending continuity of life.

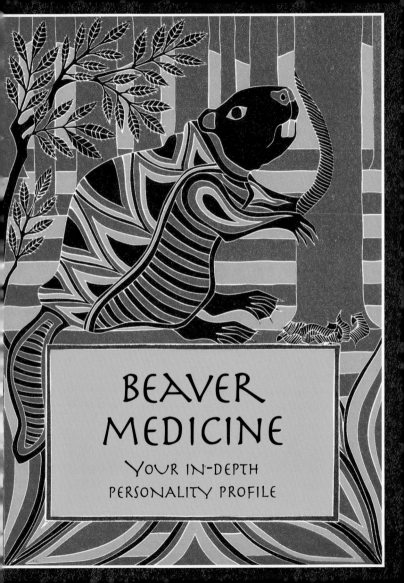

BEAVER
MEDICINE

YOUR IN-DEPTH
PERSONALITY PROFILE

SEASON OF BIRTH
GROWING TIME

THE ENERGIZING POWER OF SPRING DURING THE SECOND
BIRTH TIME OF THE SEASON LENDS THOSE BORN THEN
THE QUALITIES OF EXPANSIVENESS AND PERSISTENCE.

Growing time is one of the twelve birth times, the fundamental division of the year into twelve seasonal segments (see pp.12–13). As the middle period of the Spring cycle, it is a time of rapid growth, when roots establish themselves more securely in the earth and when flowers start to bloom. Grasses spread swiftly, transforming the landscape,

INFLUENCE OF NATURE
The qualities and characteristics imbued in Nature at this time form the basis of your own nature. So, just as Spring is reaching its height, if you were born during Growing time you too will possess an expansive, "earthy" nature. You express the need inherent in Nature at this time simultaneously to establish firm roots and to go out into the world. You are vigorous in defending both your security and the right to pursue your desires and ambitions. You have a warm and affectionate temperament, reflecting the growing warmth of the Sun at this time. Although, when you or someone you love is threatened, your attitude can be every bit as

chilling as a sudden Spring shower. Stability is as important to you as it is to the plant that is trying to establish itself in the earth – you cannot grow or develop without it. Consequently, your relationships tend to be long lasting, and you make a loyal partner or friend.

STAGE OF LIFE

Growing time embraces the midway point between the Spring equinox and the Summer solstice, celebrated by ancient peoples as May Day.

This festival of initiation and fertility highlights the fecundity of Nature during this time, which might be compared to the transition period from child to young adult that is marked by puberty. It is a time of life when sexual awareness develops and romantic relationships start to assume major importance.

ACHIEVE YOUR POTENTIAL

Security and contentment are important to you and you have the persistence, warmth, and tenacity to achieve much that is lasting and worthwhile at work and at home.

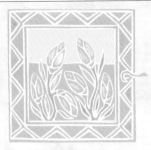

Nature's energy

Nature reaches its most rapid growth point in this, the middle cycle of Spring. Plants begin to flourish, establishing strong roots in the soil, while their flowers and leaves start to bloom and develop.

Your determination to create a stable and secure environment can turn into stubbornness, however, making you inflexible to change and inconsiderate of others' wishes.

Try to keep an open mind whatever the situation, and adapt your ambitions if circumstances change. Your expansive nature may lead you to make extravagant gestures and you have a tendency to become overly materialistic. Learn to listen to your spiritual needs, too.

"Life is a circle from childhood to childhood; so it is with everything where power moves." Black Elk teaching

BIRTH TOTEM
THE BEAVER

THE ESSENTIAL NATURE AND CHARACTERISTIC BEHAVIOUR OF THE BEAVER EXPRESSES THE PERSONALITY TYPE OF THOSE BORN DURING GROWING TIME.

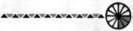

Like the beaver, people born during Growing time are methodical, reliable, industrious, and persistent. If you were born at this time, you have a practical, dependable, and affectionate nature that thrives in a secure, comfortable, and visually pleasing environment.

Constructive and hard-working, you derive much satisfaction from creating a harmonious and stable atmosphere at home and at work. Creative and dextrous, you excel at making the best of situations and mending troubled relationships. Your artistry and refined aesthetic sense is often apparent in the interior decor of your home, which you like to fill with beautiful objects.

Affectionate and consistent, you are a loyal friend and your relationships are usually enduring. However, your desire to possess valuable artefacts can sometimes extend to the desire to own the people in your life, in your need to feel materially and emotionally secure.

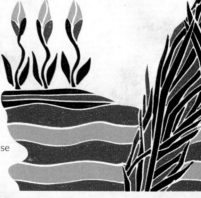

HEALTH MATTERS

Although you tend to lead a sedentary or luxurious lifestyle, you have a robust constitution that can withstand a measure of self-indulgence. You are susceptible to throat infections and suffer problems with the bladder more often than most. You may also suffer from heart or kidney problems in your later years.

Beaver power

Industrious and strong-willed, the beaver also expresses the constructive and patient aspects of the capable people born at this time.

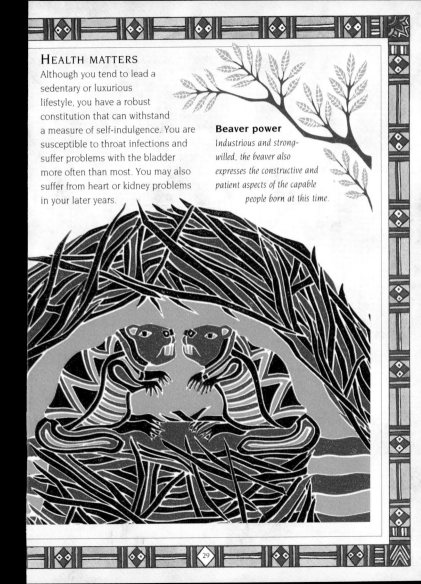

THE BEAVER AND
RELATIONSHIPS

WARM AND RELIABLE, BEAVER PEOPLE ARE LOYAL
FRIENDS. THEY MAKE COMMITTED AND LASTING
RELATIONSHIPS BUT MAY BE POSSESSIVE.

With their love of security and stability, Beaver people cherish old friends and cultivate long-standing relationships. If your birth totem is Beaver, you make a dependable friend and colleague, who enjoys working to benefit others as well as yourself. However, your desire to improve matters can make you seem controlling; if you can adopt a more flexible attitude, you will find your company more in demand.

LOVING RELATIONSHIPS

Like your totem animal, you work hard to create a secure home and harmonious environment. Highly affectionate and loyal, Beaver people often form steady, long-lasting relationships. Male Beaver is reliable and romantic, while female Beaver is a good home-maker. Both appreciate beauty and comfort, and can be highly sensual and responsive lovers.

When problems arise, it often stems from your constant need for reassurance, which can make you jealous and overbearing. Take care that your love of security does not make life with you lack excitement.

COPING WITH BEAVER

Beaver people tend to be cautious and rather rigid, so changes and new ideas should be presented to them gradually or they will feel threatened and insecure. Where they can be involved in engineering the change, they will feel more at ease. They are demanding of others and can also be self-critical, but they respond well to gentle coaxing, reassurance, and recognition of their qualities.

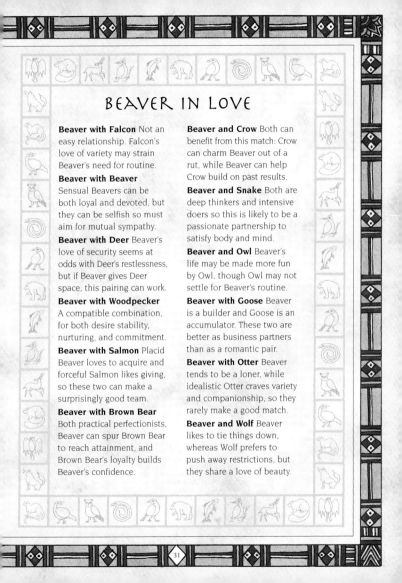

BEAVER IN LOVE

Beaver with Falcon Not an easy relationship. Falcon's love of variety may strain Beaver's need for routine.

Beaver with Beaver Sensual Beavers can be both loyal and devoted, but they can be selfish so must aim for mutual sympathy.

Beaver with Deer Beaver's love of security seems at odds with Deer's restlessness, but if Beaver gives Deer space, this pairing can work.

Beaver with Woodpecker A compatible combination, for both desire stability, nurturing, and commitment.

Beaver with Salmon Placid Beaver loves to acquire and forceful Salmon likes giving, so these two can make a surprisingly good team.

Beaver with Brown Bear Both practical perfectionists, Beaver can spur Brown Bear to reach attainment, and Brown Bear's loyalty builds Beaver's confidence.

Beaver and Crow Both can benefit from this match: Crow can charm Beaver out of a rut, while Beaver can help Crow build on past results.

Beaver and Snake Both are deep thinkers and intensive doers so this is likely to be a passionate partnership to satisfy body and mind.

Beaver and Owl Beaver's life may be made more fun by Owl, though Owl may not settle for Beaver's routine.

Beaver with Goose Beaver is a builder and Goose is an accumulator. These two are better as business partners than as a romantic pair.

Beaver with Otter Beaver tends to be a loner, while idealistic Otter craves variety and companionship, so they rarely make a good match.

Beaver and Wolf Beaver likes to tie things down, whereas Wolf prefers to push away restrictions, but they share a love of beauty.

DIRECTIONAL TOTEM
THE EAGLE

THE EAGLE SYMBOLIZES THE INFLUENCE OF THE EAST ON
BEAVER PEOPLE, WHOSE FAR-SIGHTEDNESS IS FOCUSED
ON MAKING PROVISION FOR THE FUTURE.

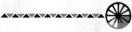

Awakening time, Growing time, and Flowering time all fall within the quarter of the Medicine Wheel associated with the East Direction or Wind.

The East is aligned with Spring and the dawn of the new day, and it is therefore associated with new beginnings, openness, illumination, and revival. The power of the East's influence is primarily with the spirit, and its principal function is the power of determining. It takes as its totem the soaring, far-sighted eagle.

The specific influence of the East on Beaver people is on putting down roots, ensuring a stable foundation for the future. It may be likened to adolescence and a growing

Eagle mask
This Tlingit shaman's headdress represents the eagle, which is associated with being far-sighted.

awareness of life – both its pleasures and its responsibilities. It is also associated with the ability to enjoy life in the present while making provision for the long-term.

EAGLE CHARACTERISTICS

The eagle can fly high in the sky, so Native Americans associated it with lofty ideals and high principles – and with illumination gained from coming closer to the spirit and the source of life. It is also a bird that can

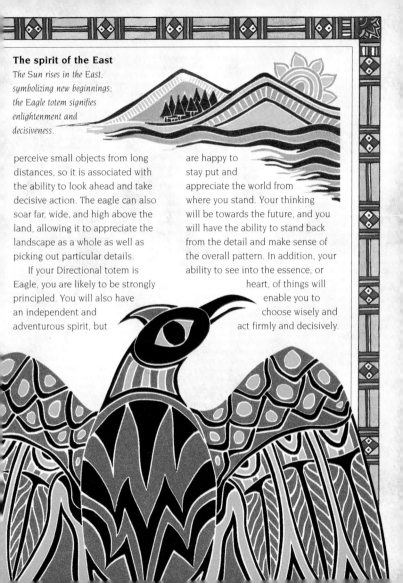

The spirit of the East

The Sun rises in the East, symbolizing new beginnings; the Eagle totem signifies enlightenment and decisiveness.

perceive small objects from long distances, so it is associated with the ability to look ahead and take decisive action. The eagle can also soar far, wide, and high above the land, allowing it to appreciate the landscape as a whole as well as picking out particular details.

If your Directional totem is Eagle, you are likely to be strongly principled. You will also have an independent and adventurous spirit, but are happy to stay put and appreciate the world from where you stand. Your thinking will be towards the future, and you will have the ability to stand back from the detail and make sense of the overall pattern. In addition, your ability to see into the essence, or heart, of things will enable you to choose wisely and act firmly and decisively.

ELEMENTAL TOTEM
THE TURTLE

LIKE THE TURTLE, WHICH TAKES LIFE ONE STEP AT A TIME, BEAVER PEOPLE'S PERSISTENT NATURE MEANS THEY ARE PATIENT IN THE PURSUIT OF THEIR GOALS.

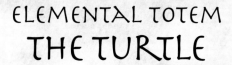

The Elemental Aspect of Beaver people is Earth. They share this Aspect with Brown Bear and Goose people, who all therefore belong to the same Elemental family or "clan" (see pp.20–21 for an introduction to the influence of the Elements).

THE TURTLE CLAN

Each Elemental clan has a totem to provide insight into its essential characteristics. The totem of the Elemental clan of Earth is Turtle, which symbolizes a persistent, careful, practical, and methodical nature with a mature outlook.

Down to Earth
The turtle symbolizes the fundamental qualities of the Element of Earth: stability and persistence.

The turtle is a gentle, slow-moving creature that progresses steadily at its own pace until it reaches its desired destination. So, if you belong to this clan, you will have a patient, tenacious, and down-to-earth personality.

Constructive and creative, you are happy to work hard, and your keen ability to focus helps you overcome obstacles to achieve your goals. You dislike disorder and may feel threatened by change. You can be inflexible and stubborn, and crave stability in order to feel at ease.

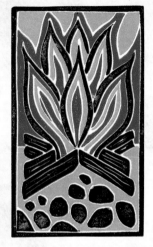

Earth of Fire

The Element of Earth feeds Fire, generating tenacity and the energy to achieve results.

You may have a tendency to be possessive and rigid, driven by the enthusiasm of Fire and the firmness and persistence of Earth. In situations where your outlook or approach is questioned or if your stability seems to be under threat, you may feel vulnerable and frustrated.

At times like these, or when you are feeling low or lacking in energy, try this revitalizing exercise. Find a quiet spot in a woodland, garden, or park, away from the polluting effects of traffic and the activities of others.

You have an instinctive affinity for the Earth and plants, so sit or stand with both feet firmly in contact with the ground, and simply notice and receive the natural beauty of growing things around you. Allow the energizing power of the life-force to refresh your body, mind, and spirit.

ELEMENTAL PROFILE

For Beaver people, the predominant Elemental Aspect of persistent Earth is fundamentally affected by the qualities of your Principal Element – vibrant Fire. Consequently, if you were born at this time, you are likely to have an abundance of creativity and enthusiasm, suffused with the energy needed to get things done.

STONE AFFINITY
BLOODSTONE

By using the gemstone with which your own essence resonates, you can tap into the power of the Earth itself and awaken your inner strengths.

Gemstones are minerals that are formed within the Earth itself in an exceedingly slow but continuous process. Native Americans valued them not only for their beauty but also for being literally part of the Earth, and therefore possessing part of its life-force. They regarded gemstones as being "alive" – channellers of energy that could be used in many ways: to heal, to protect, or for meditation.

Every gemstone has a different energy or vibration. On the Medicine Wheel, a stone is associated with each birth time, the energy of which resonates with the essence of those

Polished bloodstone

Bloodstone is also known as heliotrope, which means "sun-reflecting". It is thought to lift the energies towards the spiritual Sun.

born during that time. Because of this energy affiliation, your gemstone can help bring you into harmony with the Earth and create balance within yourself. It can develop your good qualities and endow you with the abilities you need.

ENERGY RESONANCE

Beaver people have an affinity with bloodstone – a form of chalcedony that is green with flecks of red. Like plants that reach upwards for the Sun, so the green of this stone is believed to have uplifting qualities. It can help to stimulate and align energy in the body. Native

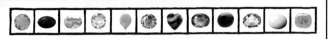

ACTIVATE YOUR GEMSTONE

Obtain a piece of bloodstone and cleanse it by holding it under cold running water. Allow it to dry naturally, then, holding the stone with both hands, bring it up to your mouth and blow into it sharply and hard three or four times in order to impregnate it with your breath. Next, hold it firmly in one hand and silently welcome it into your life as a friend and helper.

When you feel out of balance or want to restore outer or inner harmony, use the bloodstone to help you meditate. Find a quiet spot to sit without fear of interruption and take the piece of bloodstone in your left hand to receive its energies. Focus your thoughts on the problem and, with the help of your affinity stone, seek a solution. Listen for the still, quiet voice of your inner self.

Americans believed it could bring balance and harmony to the body's power centres and also alleviate certain blood-related disorders.

If your birth totem is Beaver, you will find bloodstone helpful in reducing your levels of stress and anxiety. It can also be powerful in strengthening bonds in relationships and friendships, enhancing your own intrinsic aptitude for bringing harmony into difficult situations, and mending discord between friends and colleagues.

Bloodstone power
To benefit most from its effect, wear bloodstone as a ring or brooch, or carry a piece of it in a small, protective pouch.

"The outline of the stone is round; the power of the stone is endless." Lakota Sioux teaching

TREE AFFINITY
ROWAN

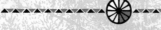

GAIN A DEEPER UNDERSTANDING OF YOUR OWN NATURE
AND AWAKEN POWERS LYING DORMANT WITHIN YOU BY
RESPECTING AND CONNECTING WITH YOUR AFFINITY TREE.

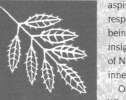

Trees have an important part to play in the protection of Nature's mechanisms and in the maintenance of the Earth's atmospheric balance, which is essential for the survival of the human race.

Native Americans referred to trees as "Standing People" because they stand firm, obtaining strength from their connection with the Earth. They therefore teach us the importance of being grounded, whilst at the same time listening to, and reaching for, our higher aspirations. When respected as living beings, trees can provide insight into the workings of Nature and our own inner selves.

On the Medicine Wheel, each birth time is associated with a particular kind of tree, the basic qualities of which complement the nature of those born during that time. Beaver people have an affinity with the rowan. A tough, adaptable tree, the rowan was regarded as a protector of earth energy – the Beaver's principal element. It was thought to guard against misfortune

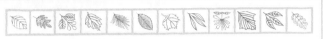

CONNECT WITH YOUR TREE

Appreciate the beauty of your affinity tree and study its nature carefully, for it has an affinity with your own nature.

The rowan is a small tree, tougher than its delicate appearance suggests, which can grow almost anywhere. It thrives in high altitudes so is also known as the mountain ash. Clusters of creamy flowers are followed by generous masses of red berries.

Try the following exercise when you need to revitalize your inner strength. Stand beside your affinity tree. Place the palms of your hands on its trunk and rest your forehead on the backs of your hands. Inhale slowly and let energy from the tree's roots flow through your body. If easily available, obtain a cutting or twig from your affinity tree to keep as a totem or helper.

and evil so was often grown on sacred sites or next to homes. The well-being of Beaver people often relies on a sense of security. When feeling insecure, Beaver people can tap into the rowan's powers of protection by connecting with their tree (see panel above).

HIGHER PLANES

If your birth totem is Beaver, you are generous and tenacious, but can also be set in your ways, limiting your potential. Like the rowan, which can flourish in all kinds of situations, learn to develop a more flexible approach. The ability to adapt and a readiness to explore untried ground will bring you greater fulfilment.

The rowan's association with high places also links with the "higher" plane of creativity and inspiration. When you feel bogged down by earthly practicalities, draw on the rowan to release your creativity and to express it with greater freedom.

"All healing plants are given by Wakan-Tanka; therefore they are holy." Lakota Sioux teaching

COLOUR AFFINITY
YELLOW

ENHANCE YOUR POSITIVE QUALITIES BY USING THE
POWER OF YOUR AFFINITY COLOUR TO AFFECT YOUR
EMOTIONAL AND MENTAL STATES.

Each birth time has an affinity with a particular colour. This is the colour that resonates best with the energies of the people born during that time, expressing their essential temperament. Exposure to your affinity colour will encourage a positive emotional and mental response, while exposure to colours that clash with your affinity colour will have a negative effect on your sense of well-being.

Yellow resonates with Beaver people. Yellow is the colour of confidence, optimism, and sponaneity. It is associated with the mind and the development of the imagination, suggesting creativity and the desire to enjoy life to the full. It is a bright, cheerful colour which invigorates and enlivens,

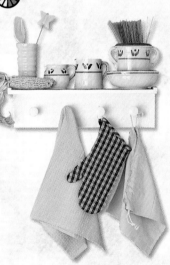

Colour scheme
Let a yellow colour theme be the thread that runs through your home, from the table settings to the walls and floors.

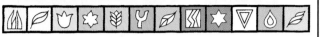

MEDITATE ON YOUR COLOUR

Place some yellow flowers – daffodils, tulips, freesias, chrysanthemums – in a yellow vase. Take the vase to a room in which you will not be disturbed for half an hour, and place the vase on a table. Sit at the table and face the flowers.

Focus your attention on the bright yellow blooms. Relax your body and concentrate your mind on the colour. This will help you to clear your mind of distractions. If a difficult situation or problem confronts you at the moment, meditate upon it. Allow any thoughts and sensations to flow through your mind and body: experience and reflect on them.

encouraging perseverance and tenacity in the face of setbacks or disappointments. Yellow also stimulates enthusiasm to take on new challenges, especially those requiring a competitive drive in order to succeed.

COLOUR BENEFITS

Strengthen your aura and enhance your positive qualities by introducing shades of yellow – primrose, buttercup, lemon – to the interior decor of your home. Spots of colour can make all the difference. A yellow lampshade, for example, can alter the ambience of a room, or try placing yellow cushions on chairs and sofas.

If you need a confidence boost, wear something that contains yellow. Whenever your energies are low, practise the colour meditation exercise outlined above to balance your emotions, awaken your creativity, and help you to feel joyful.

"The power of the spirit should be honoured with its colour." **Lakota Sioux teaching**

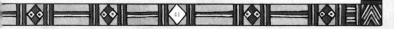

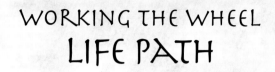

WORKING THE WHEEL
LIFE PATH

CONSIDER YOUR BIRTH PROFILE AS A STARTING POINT IN
THE DEVELOPMENT OF YOUR CHARACTER AND THE
ACHIEVEMENT OF PERSONAL FULFILMENT.

ach of the twelve birth times is associated with a particular path of learning, or with a collection of lessons to be learned through life. By following your path of learning you will develop strengths in place of weaknesses, achieve a greater sense of harmony with the world, and discover inner peace.

YOUR PATH OF LEARNING
For Beaver people, the first lesson on your path of learning is to cultivate a

more flexible approach to life. Because of your need for security you tend to hold on to attitudes or relationships from which you no longer derive any benefit, or which actively cause you harm. You would rather stick with what you know, even if it makes you unhappy, than contemplate change. Try to overcome this fear of change and give an honest reappraisal of your most

"Each man's road is shown to him within his own heart. There he sees all the truths of life." Cheyenne teaching

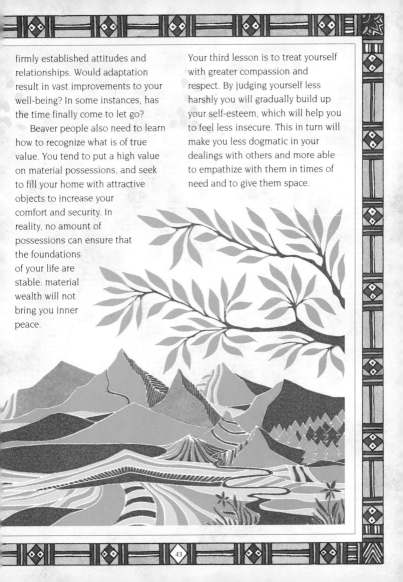

firmly established attitudes and relationships. Would adaptation result in vast improvements to your well-being? In some instances, has the time finally come to let go?

Beaver people also need to learn how to recognize what is of true value. You tend to put a high value on material possessions, and seek to fill your home with attractive objects to increase your comfort and security. In reality, no amount of possessions can ensure that the foundations of your life are stable: material wealth will not bring you inner peace.

Your third lesson is to treat yourself with greater compassion and respect. By judging yourself less harshly you will gradually build up your self-esteem, which will help you to feel less insecure. This in turn will make you less dogmatic in your dealings with others and more able to empathize with them in times of need and to give them space.

WORKING THE WHEEL
MEDICINE POWER

HARNESS THE POWERS OF OTHER BIRTH TIMES TO
TRANSFORM YOUR WEAKNESSES INTO STRENGTHS AND
MEET THE CHALLENGES IN YOUR LIFE.

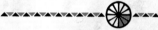

The whole spectrum of human qualities and abilities is represented on the Medicine Wheel. The totems and affinities associated with each birth time indicate the basic qualities with which those born at that time are equipped.

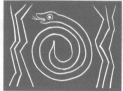

Complementary affinity
A key strength of Snake – weak in Beaver – is the ability to adapt to new circumstances.

Study your path of learning (see pp.42–43) to identify those aspects of your personality that may need to be strengthened, then look at other birth times to discover the totems and affinities that will assist you in this task. For example, your Elemental profile is Earth of Fire (see pp.34–35), so for balance you need the freedom and clarity of Air

and the adaptive qualities of Water. Otter's Elemental profile is Air of Air and Wolf's is Water of Air, so meditate on these birth totems. In addition, you may find it useful to study the profiles of the other two members of your Elemental clan of Turtle – Brown Bear and Goose – to discover how the same Elemental Aspect can be expressed differently.

Also helpful is the birth totem that sits opposite yours on the Medicine Wheel, which usually contains qualities that complement or enhance your own. This is known as your complementary affinity, which for Beaver people is Snake.

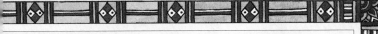

ESSENTIAL STRENGTHS

Described below are the essential strengths of each birth totem. To develop a quality that is weak in yourself or that you need to meet a particular challenge, meditate upon the birth totem that contains the attribute you need. Obtain a representation of the relevant totem – a claw, tooth, or feather; a picture, ring, or model. Affirm that the power it represents is within you.

Falcon medicine is the power of keen observation and the ability to act decisively and energetically whenever action is required.

Beaver medicine is the ability to think creatively and laterally – to develop alternative ways of doing or thinking about things.

Deer medicine is characterized by sensitivity to the intentions of others and to that which might be detrimental to your well-being.

Woodpecker medicine is the ability to establish a steady rhythm throughout life and to be tenacious in protecting all that you hold dear.

Salmon medicine is the strength to be determined and courageous in the choice of goals you want to achieve, and to have enough stamina to see a task through to the end.

Brown Bear medicine is the ability to be resourceful, hardworking, and dependable in times of need and to draw on inner strength.

Crow medicine is the ability to transform negative or non-productive situations into positive ones and to transcend limitations.

Snake medicine is the talent to adapt easily to changes in circumstances and to manage transitional phases well.

Owl medicine is the power to see clearly during times of uncertainty and to conduct life consistently, according to long-term plans.

Goose medicine is the courage to do whatever might be necessary to protect your ideals and adhere to your principles in life.

Otter medicine is the ability to connect with your inner child, to be innovative and idealistic, and to thoroughly enjoy the ordinary tasks and routines of everyday life.

Wolf medicine is the courage to act according to your intuition and instincts rather than your intellect, and to be compassionate.

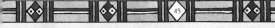

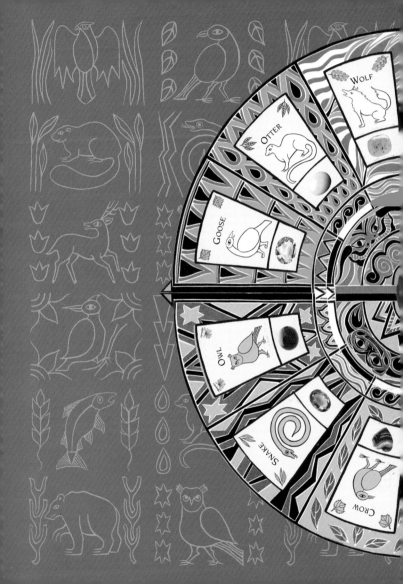